Sometimes Mommy Falls

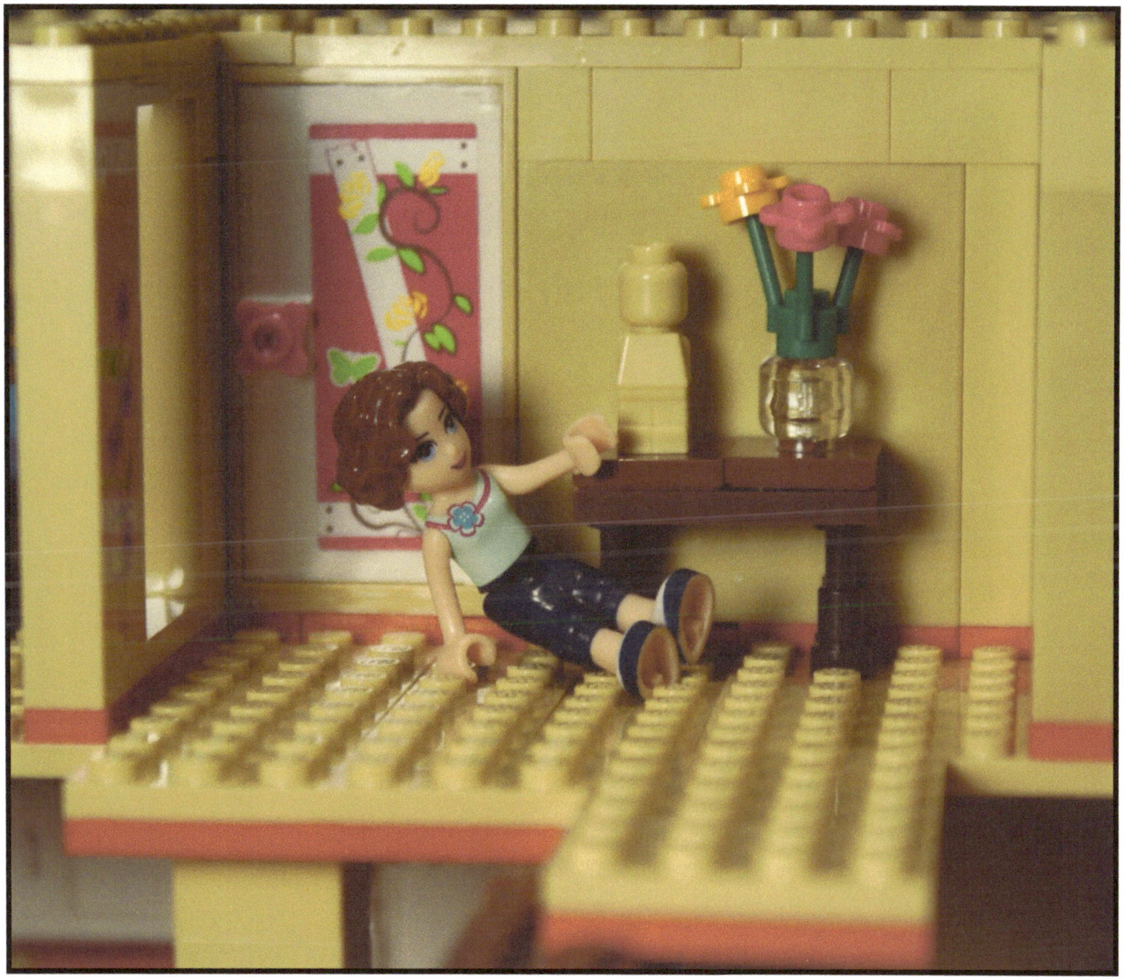

A Book About Narcolepsy and Cataplexy

To my Mom,

You are the strongest woman I know. Thank you for everything!

To my best friend Amanda[2],

You can read my mind, so you already know.

This book should not be used in any way as a means to diagnose Narcolepsy or Cataplexy. Diagnosis of any medical condition should only be made by a licensed physician.

Sometimes Mommy Falls

A Book About Narcolepsy and Cataplexy

Amanda Stock

astock204@gmail.com

ISBN-13: 978-1519132215

ISBN-10: 1519132212

First Edition 2015

This book is in no way authorized, sponsored, or endorsed by The LEGO Company

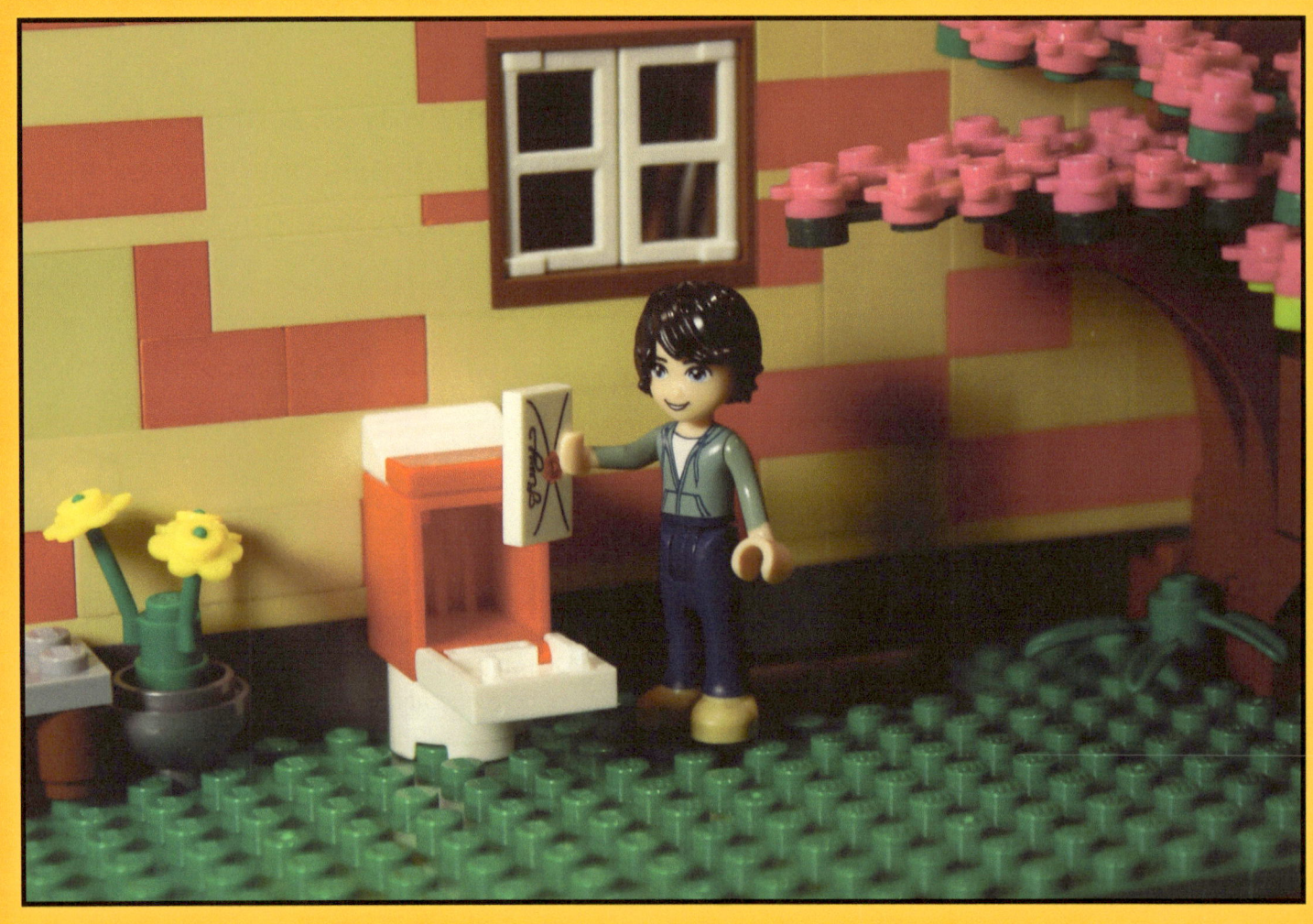

Hi! My name is Dylan.

I am so excited my mom is coming today! She hasn't made it to my last few games because she was stuck in bed. My mom has a sleep disorder called Narcolepsy.

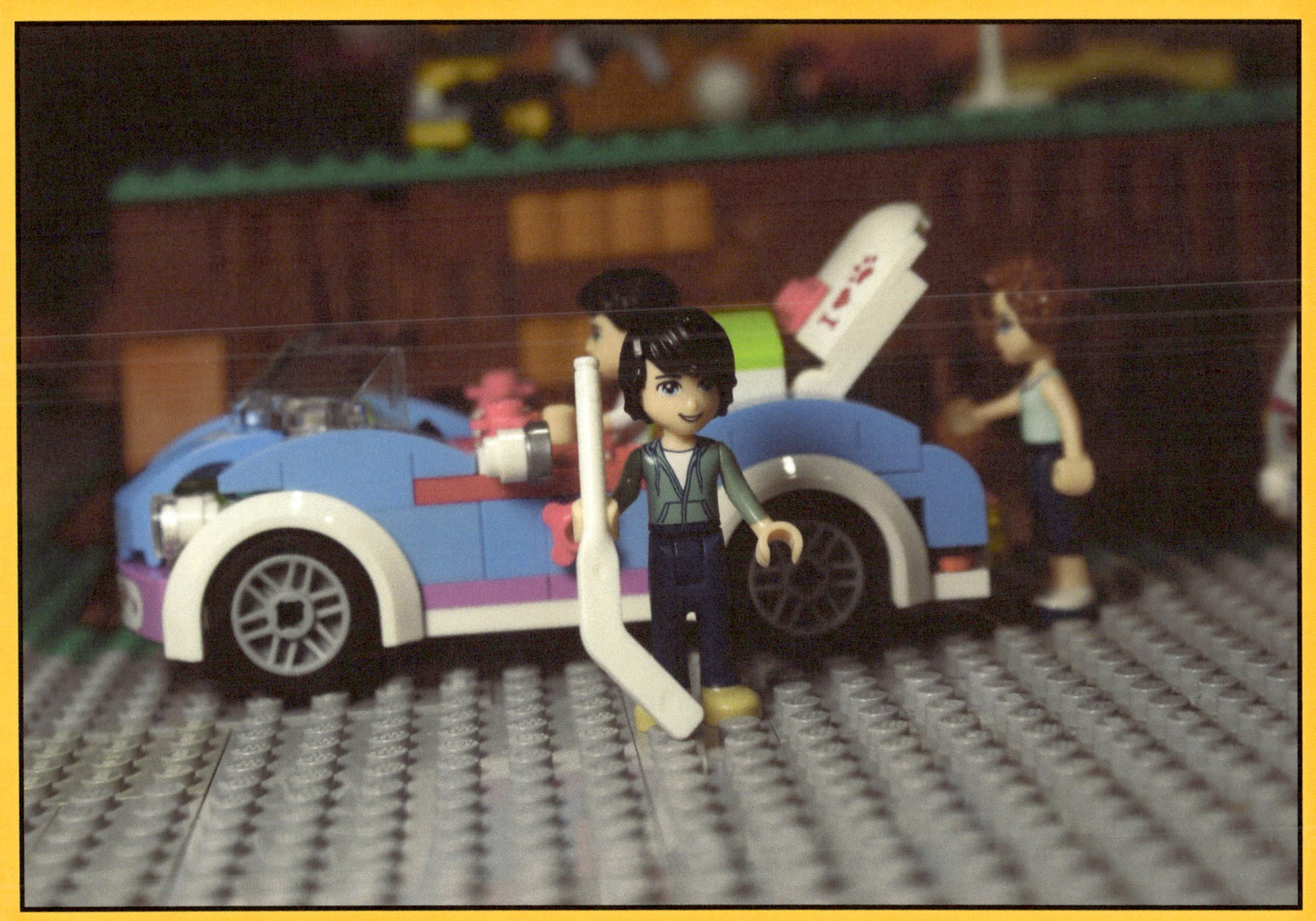

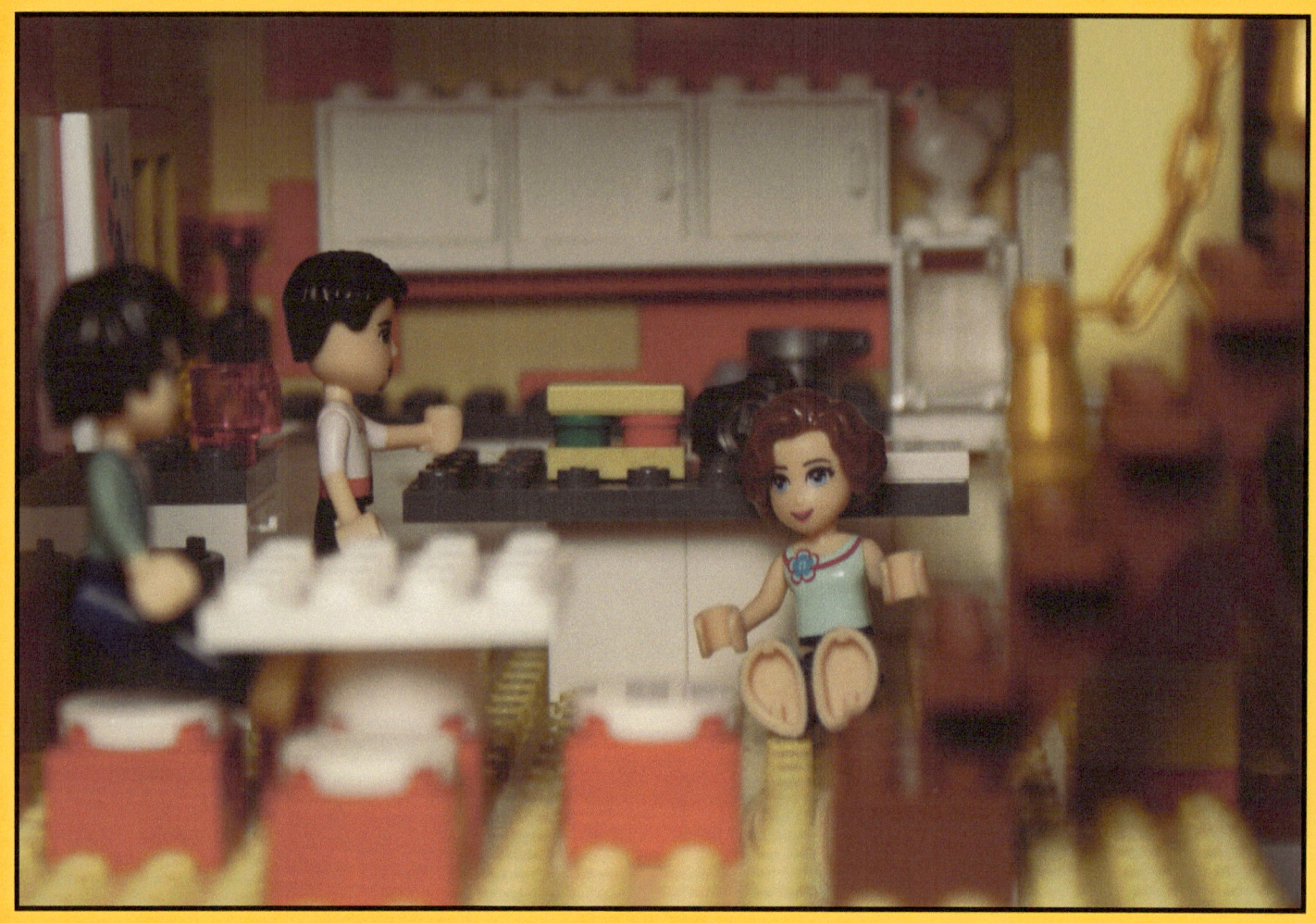

Narcolepsy makes the people who have it tired all the time, but that's not all it does. Some people, like my mom, also have Cataplexy. My parents told me to think of it like her muscles are falling asleep with out permission.

Cataplexy can make my mom's whole body sleepy or just parts of it. Sometimes she drops her pencil or can not pick something up and she gets really mad.

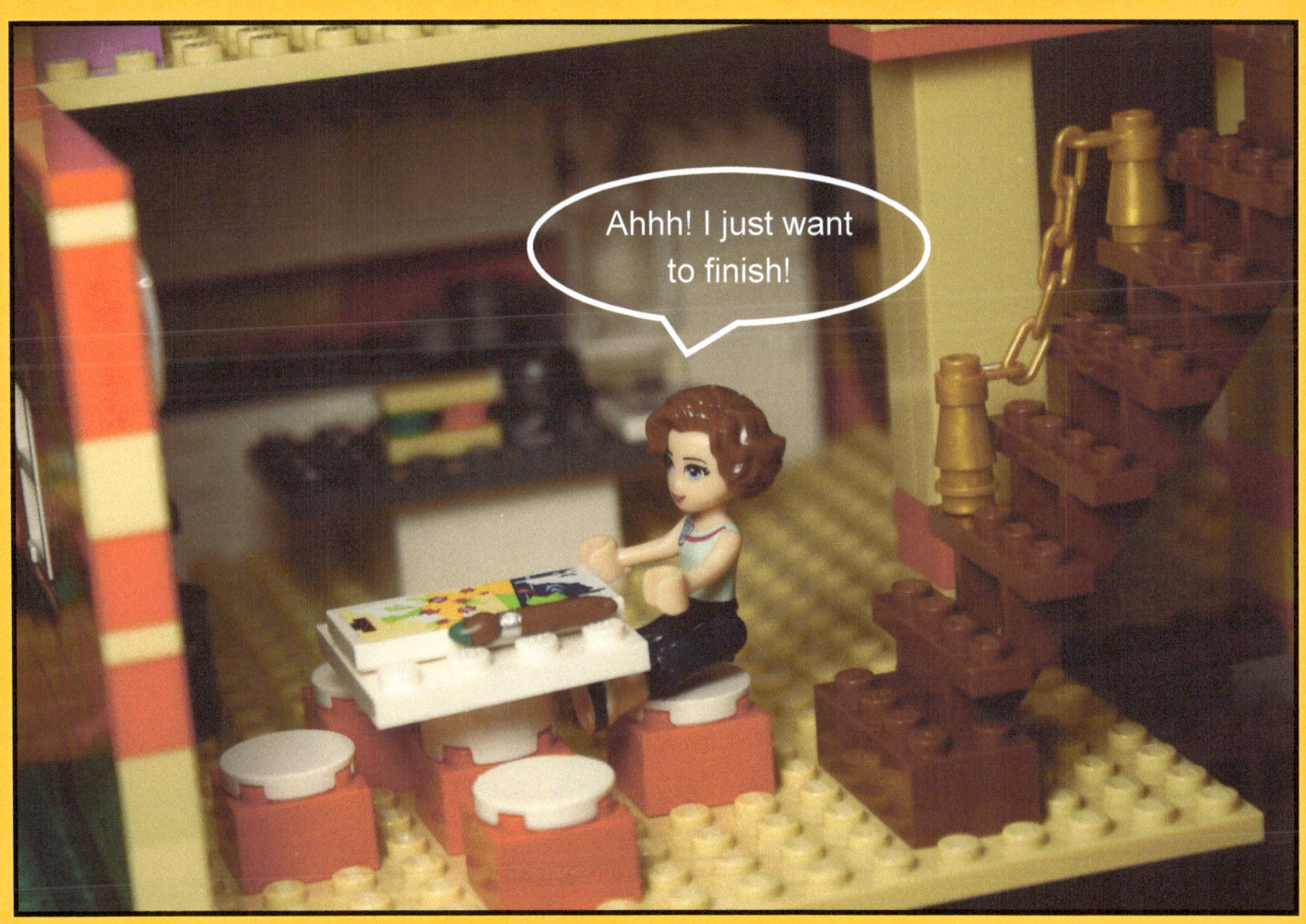

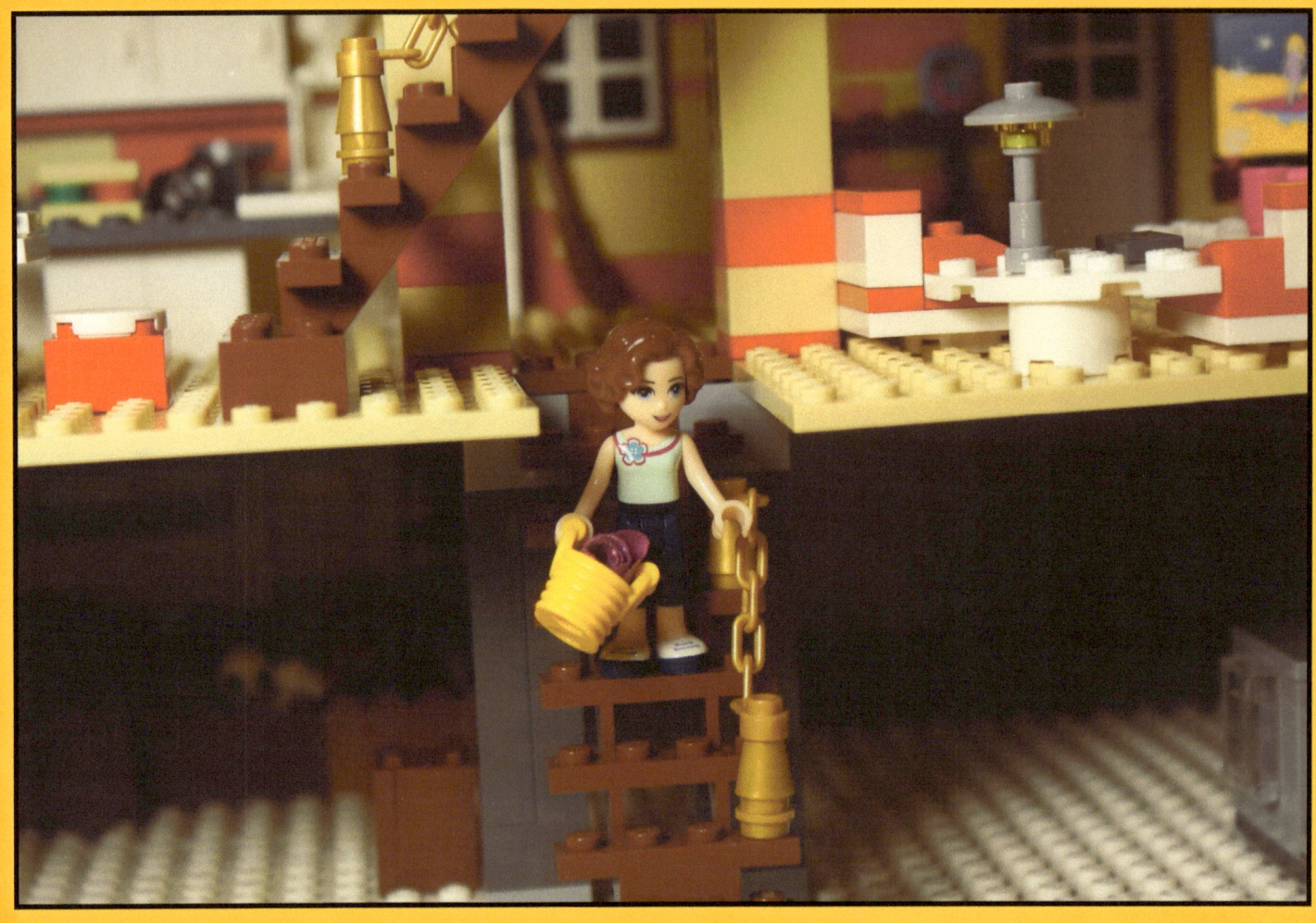

She has to be careful going down the stairs because her knees might give out on her. Stairs can be very scary for people with Cataplexy.

The worst is when her whole body gets too tired and she falls to the floor. Daddy does his best to catch her. We don't try to wake her up when it happens, we just put a pillow under her head and sit with her until she can sit up. It's scary but I know she is ok.

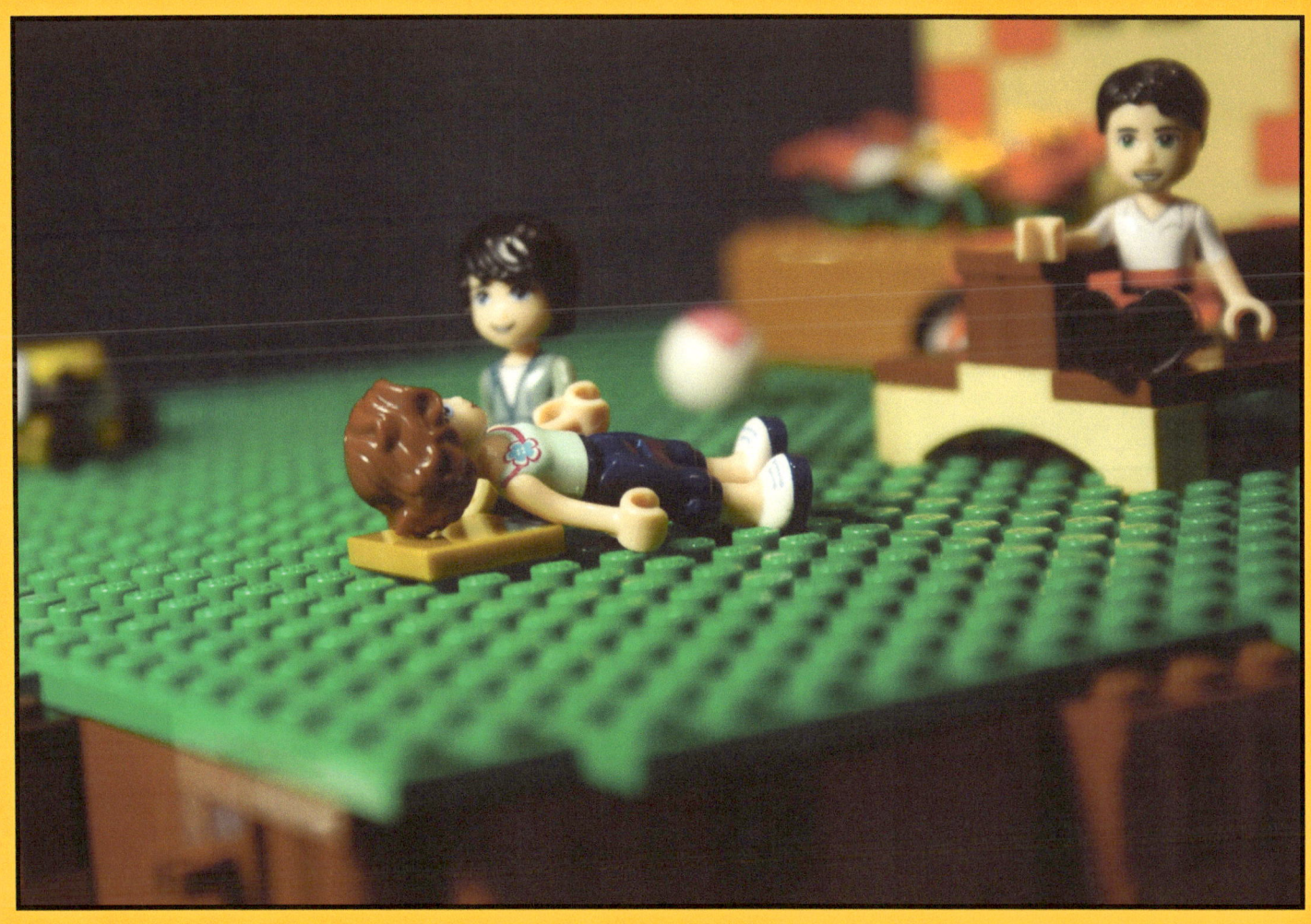

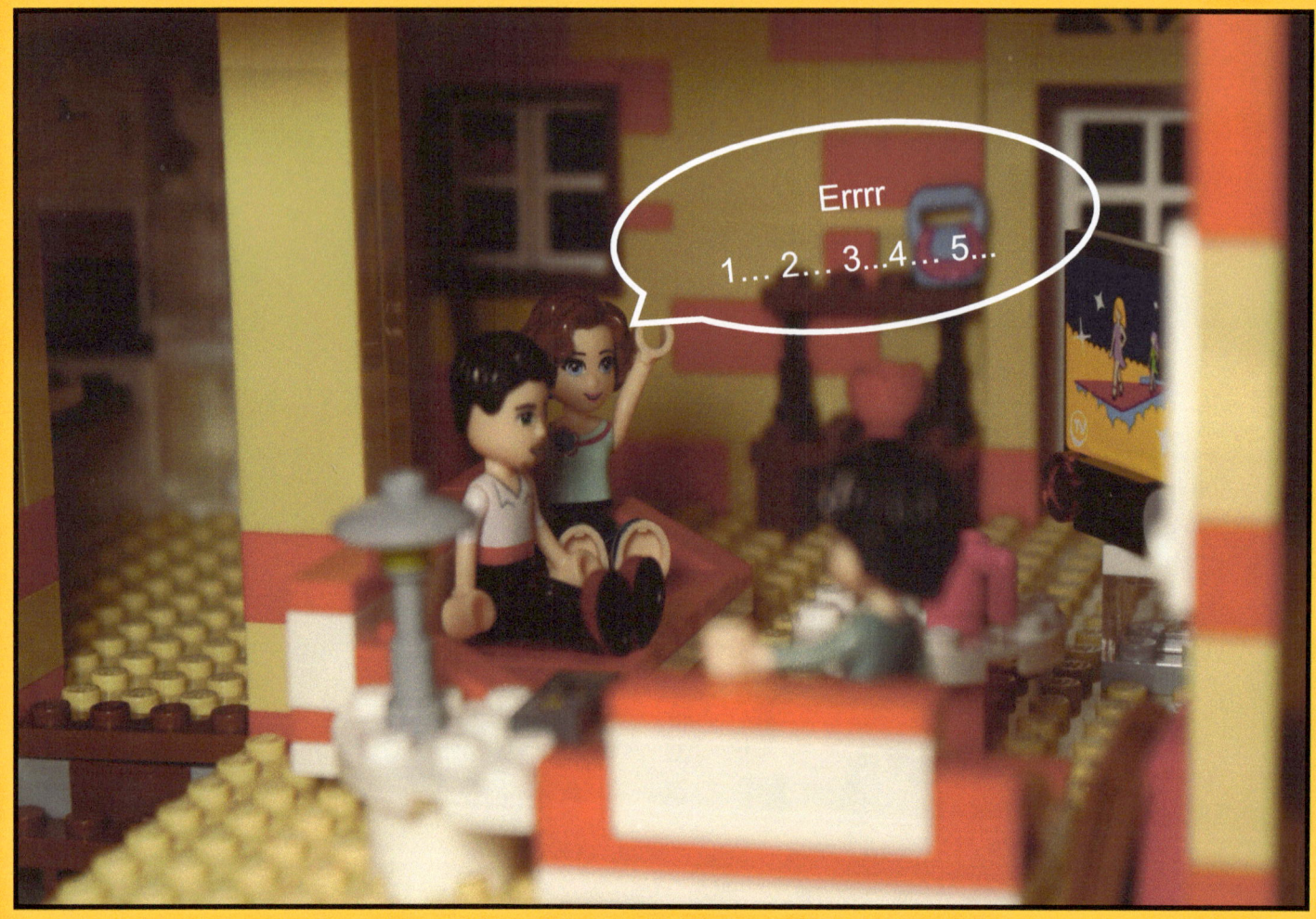

Sometimes when mom speaks her words turn into funny noises. She starts a sentence but she can't finish it, this makes her very upset and frustrated. She takes a deep breath then counts to five and most of the time she is ok again.

There are people with Narcolepsy and Cataplexy who are lucky enough to be able to drive. Sadly my mom isn't one of them. If she had an attack while driving she could hurt herself and other people. So my Dad or Grandpa take me to hockey practice and games.

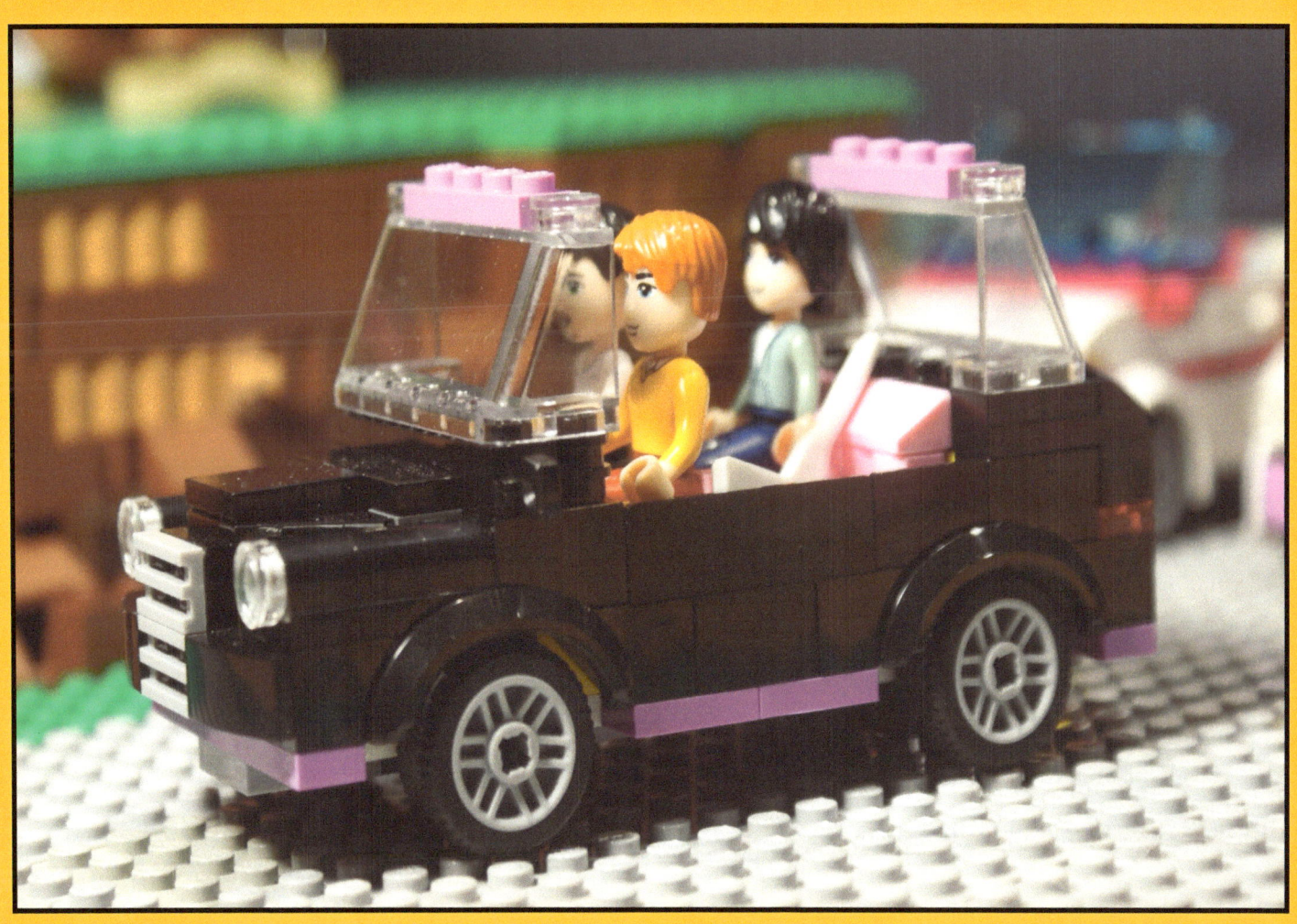

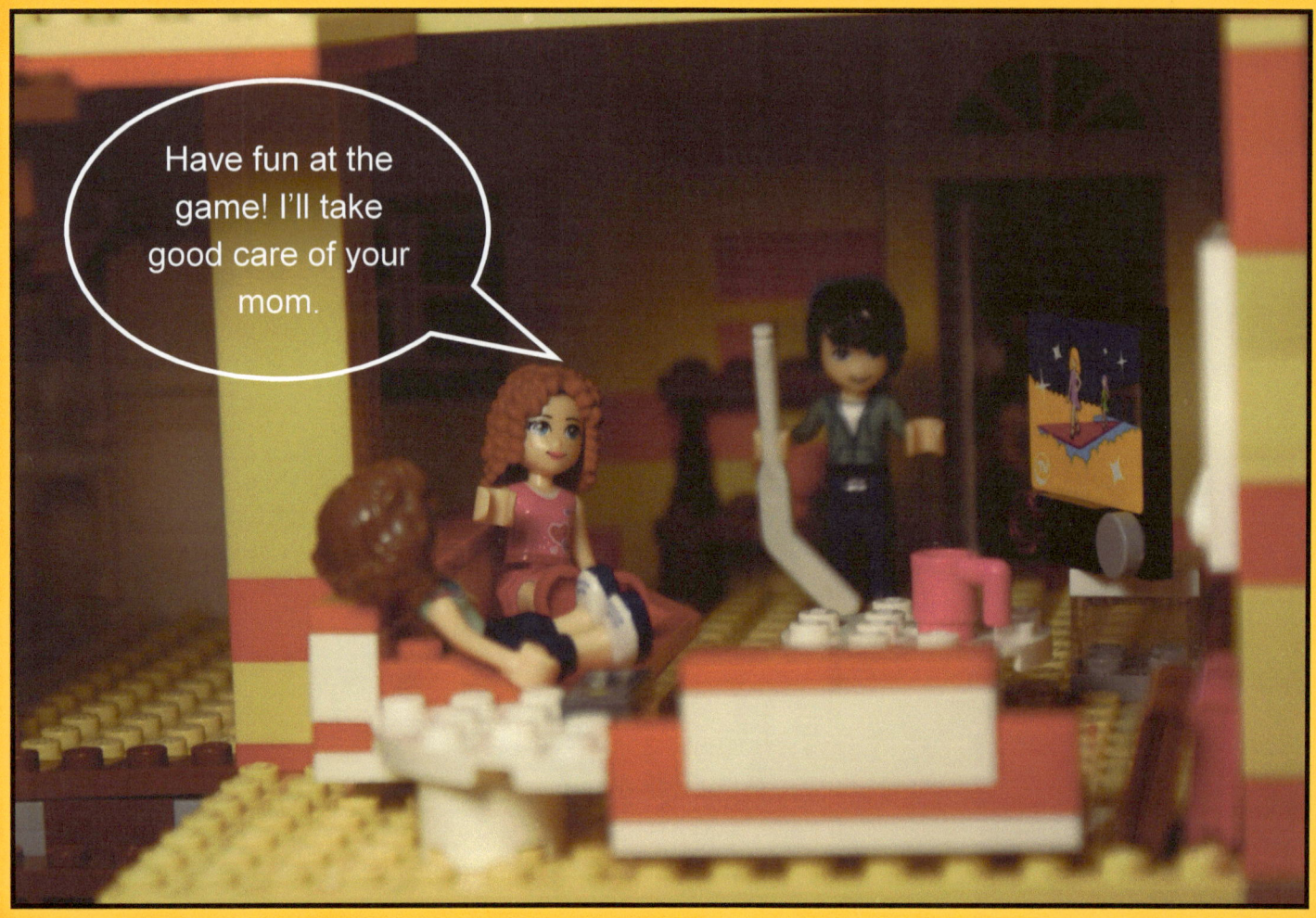

Mom tries her best to make it to my games but sometimes she is just too tired and it is hard for her to move. I really like it when she can come cheer me on. It makes me sad when she is sick and has to stay home.

My mom has to take special medication to keep her awake; she also has to take other medication to keep the Cataplexy away. It took a long time to figure out which medications worked best. Some of them made her very sick or made her symptoms worse!

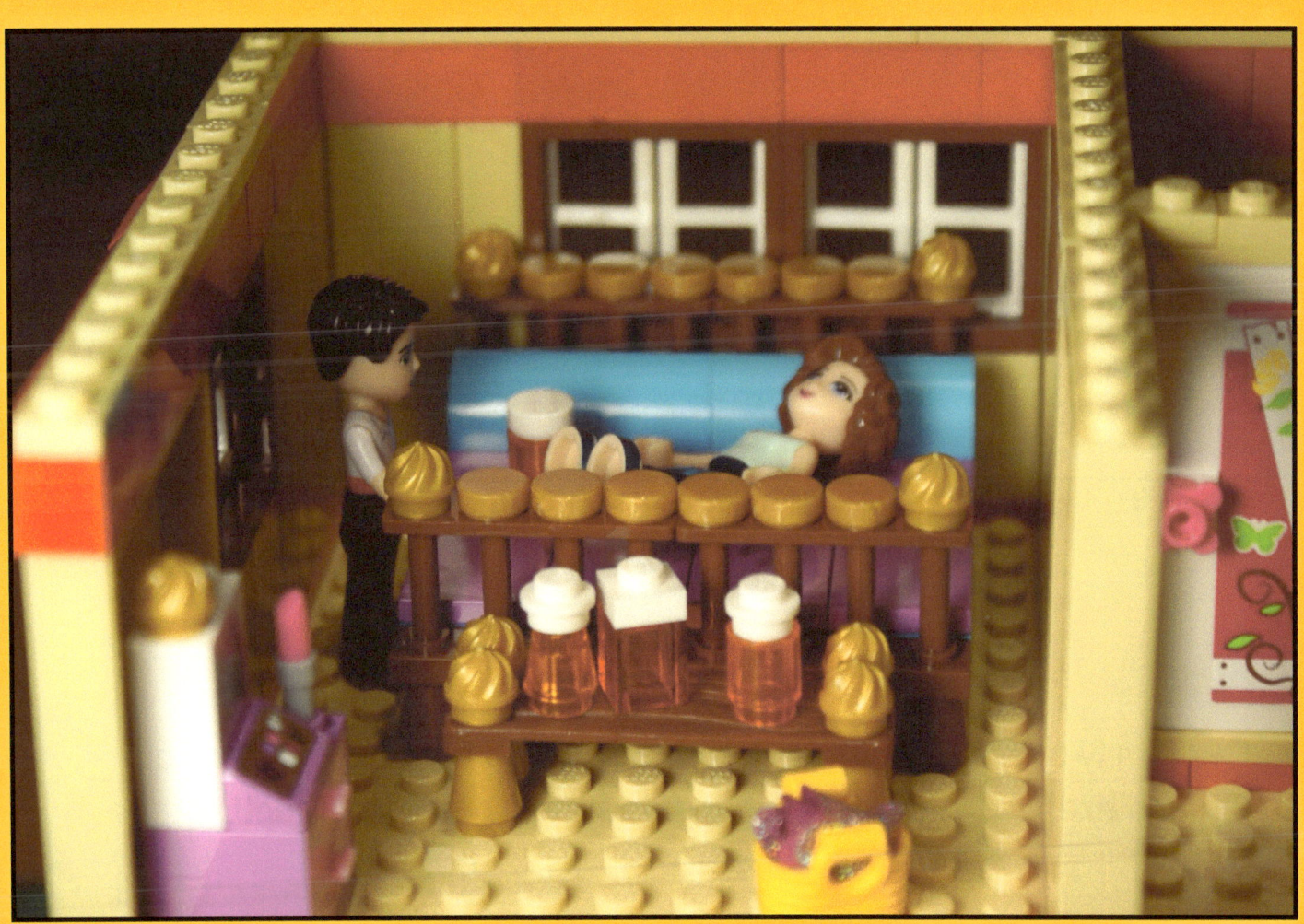

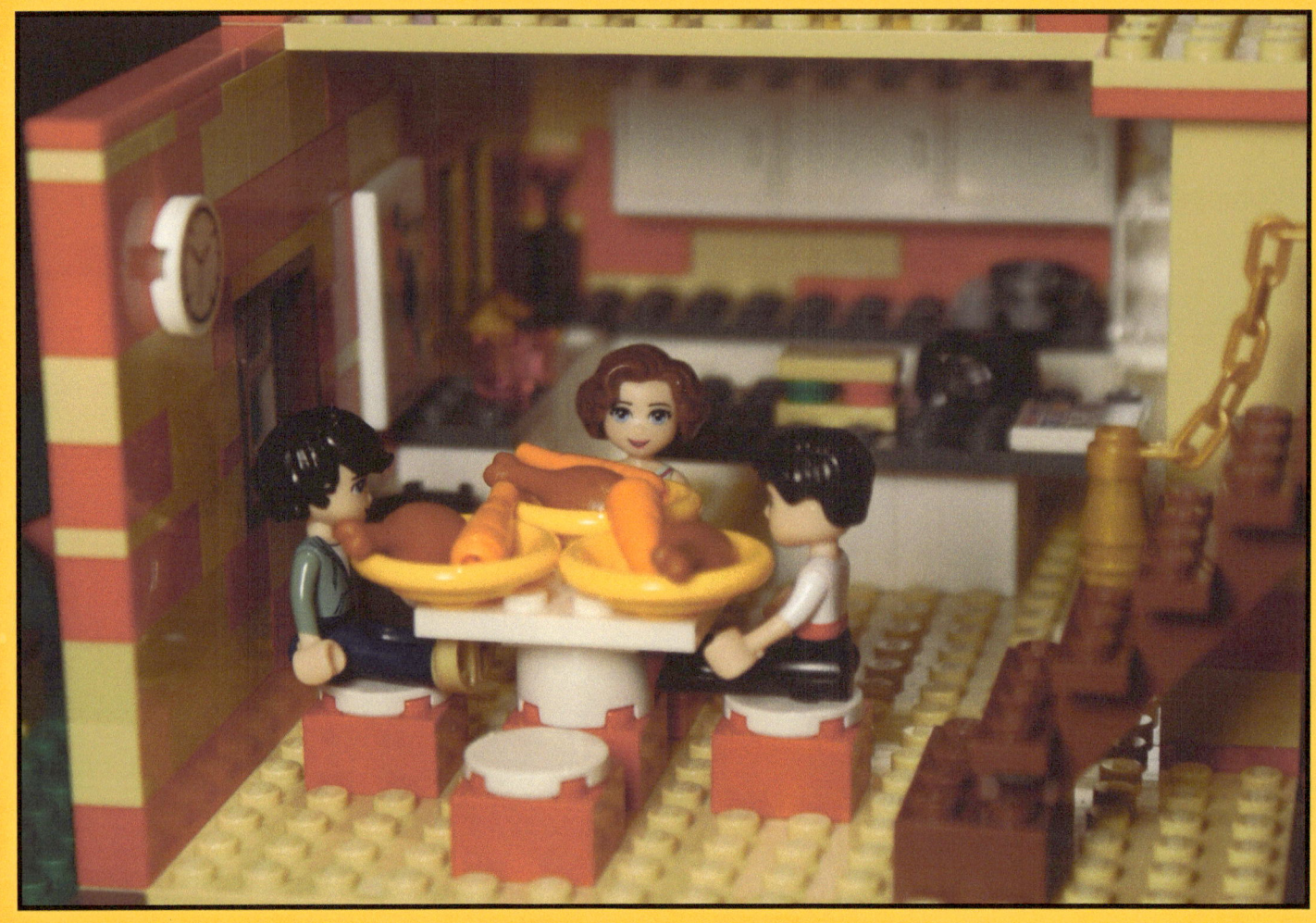

Our family tries to always eat very healthy. It's hard for my mom but she tries to exercise when she has the energy. It makes her feel better and puts a smile on her face.

She also has a bed time, just like me. She told me that keeping a regular bed time and napping the same time every day helps keep the Narcolepsy away.

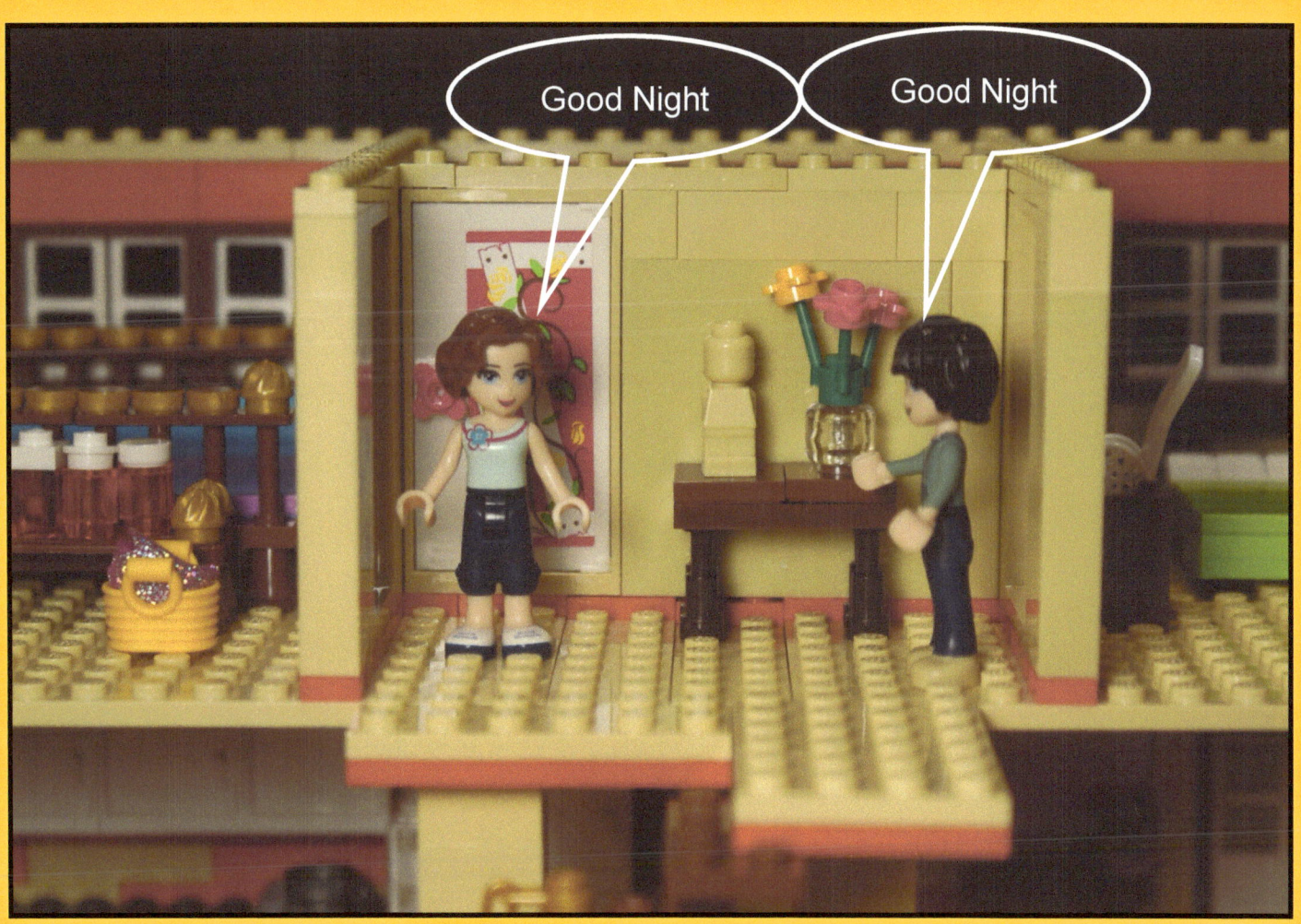

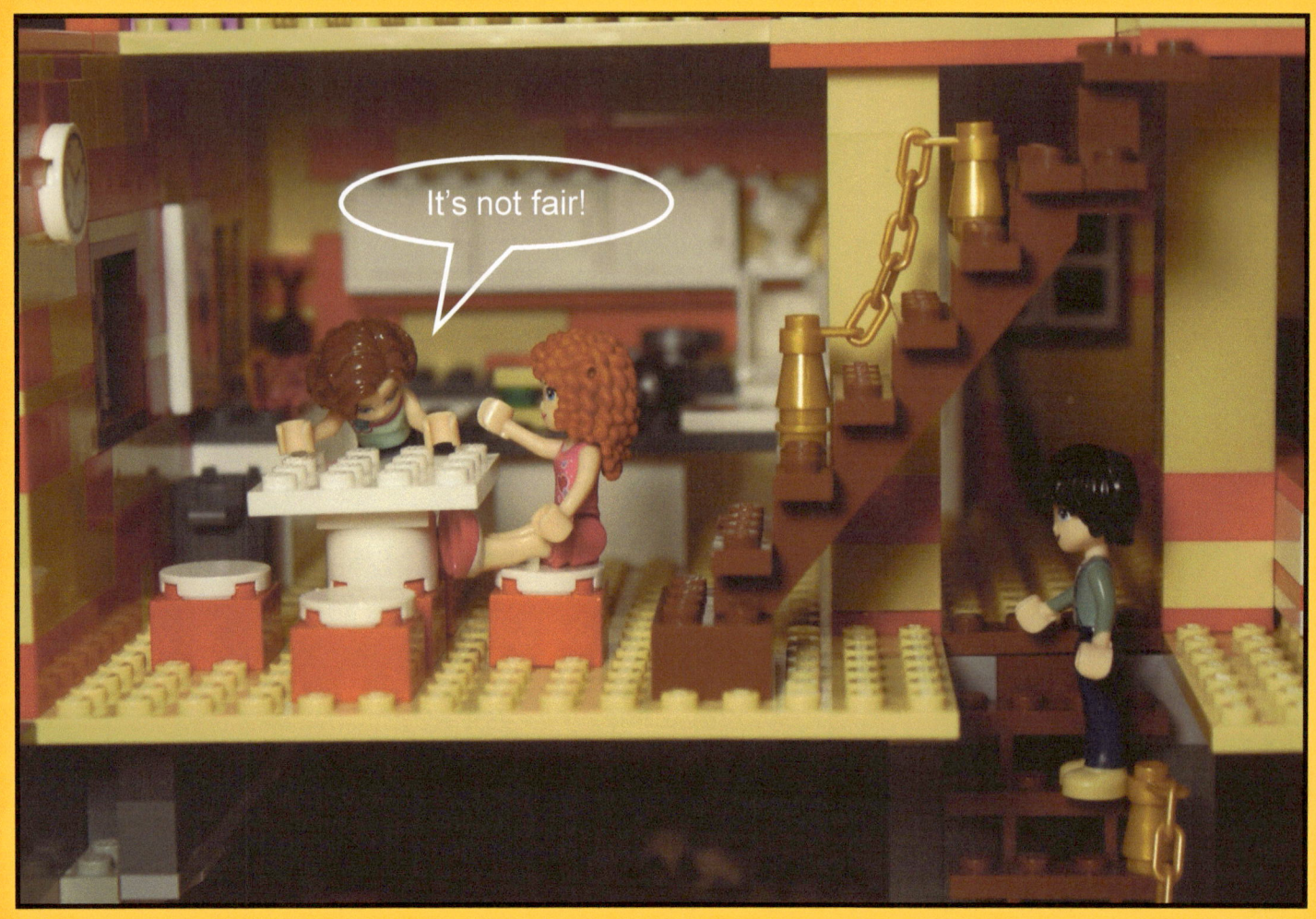

She doesn't like that her Narcolepsy can be so scary for me. Once I heard her tell her friend, "I just wish I wasn't so tired. I just want to feel normal and do what everyone else can do. I hate this."

I wish my mom could do more with me but she is still the best mom in the whole world. We make crafts together, read books, watch movies and other fun quiet activities. Even though things can be harder for her than for most people she always tries her best.

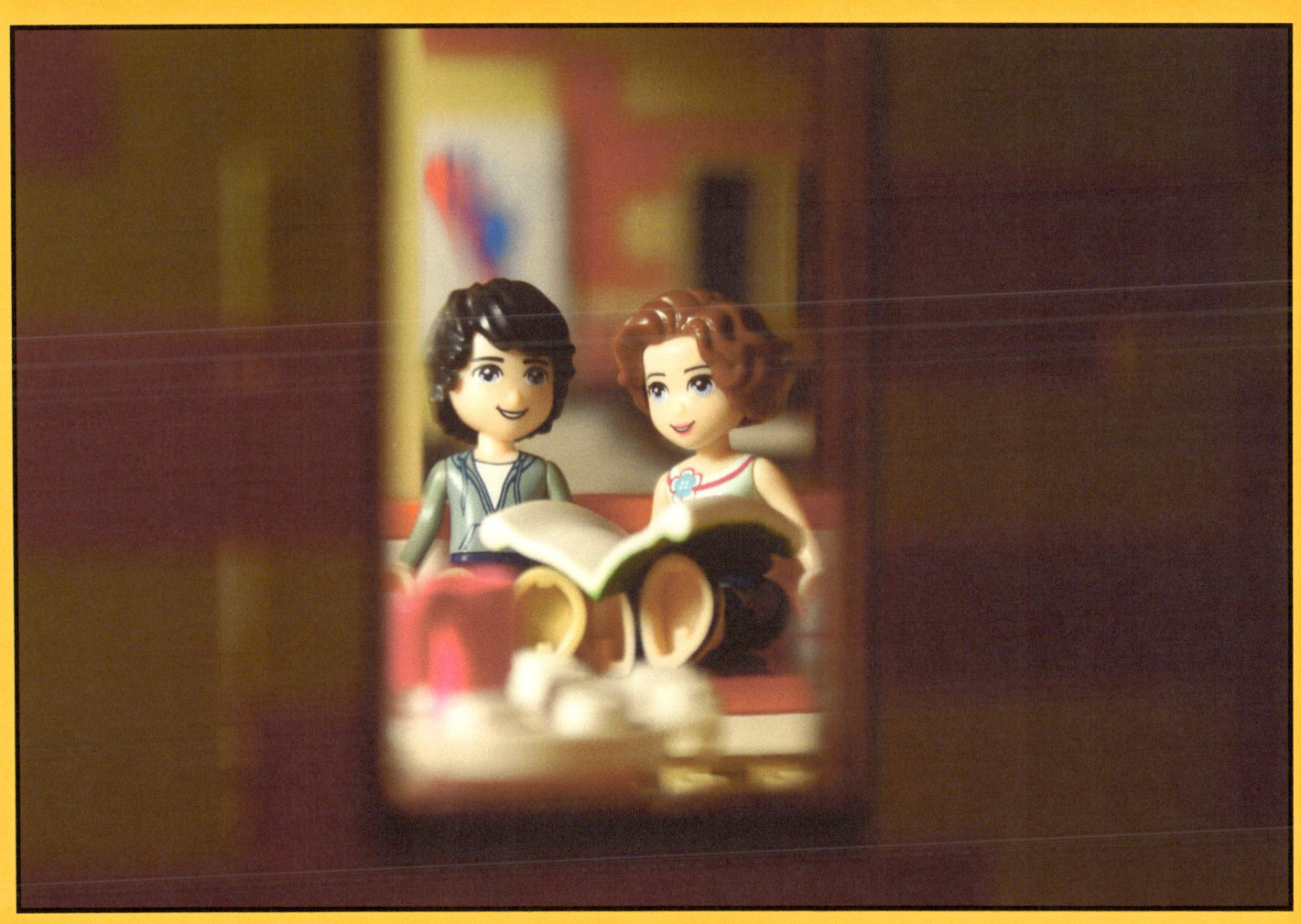

Follow up questions

- What was your favorite part of the book?
- Did the book remind you of _____?

  Person in your life with Narcolepsy

- What things in the book reminded you of _____?

  Person in your life with Narcolepsy

- Does anything in the book bother you?
- Is there anything else you would like to learn about Narcolepsy and Cataplexy

Definitions

- Sleep Disorder: When a person's sleep patterns are different then they should be
- Narcolepsy: When the brain goes sleep during times the person should be awake
- Cataplexy: Muscle weakness while someone is awake usually because of strong emotions
- Symptom: When a person does something "weird" or different that lets them or others know they might be sick.

Books in the Talking to Kids About Narcolepsy Series

Book 1 - Automatic Behavior: Sometimes My Socks are in the Freezer

Book 2 - Excessive Daytime Sleepiness: My Dad Naps Too!

Book 3 - Cataplexy: Sometimes Mommy Falls

Coming Soon!

Book 4 - Sleep Paralysis

Book 5 - Hypnagogic Hallucinations

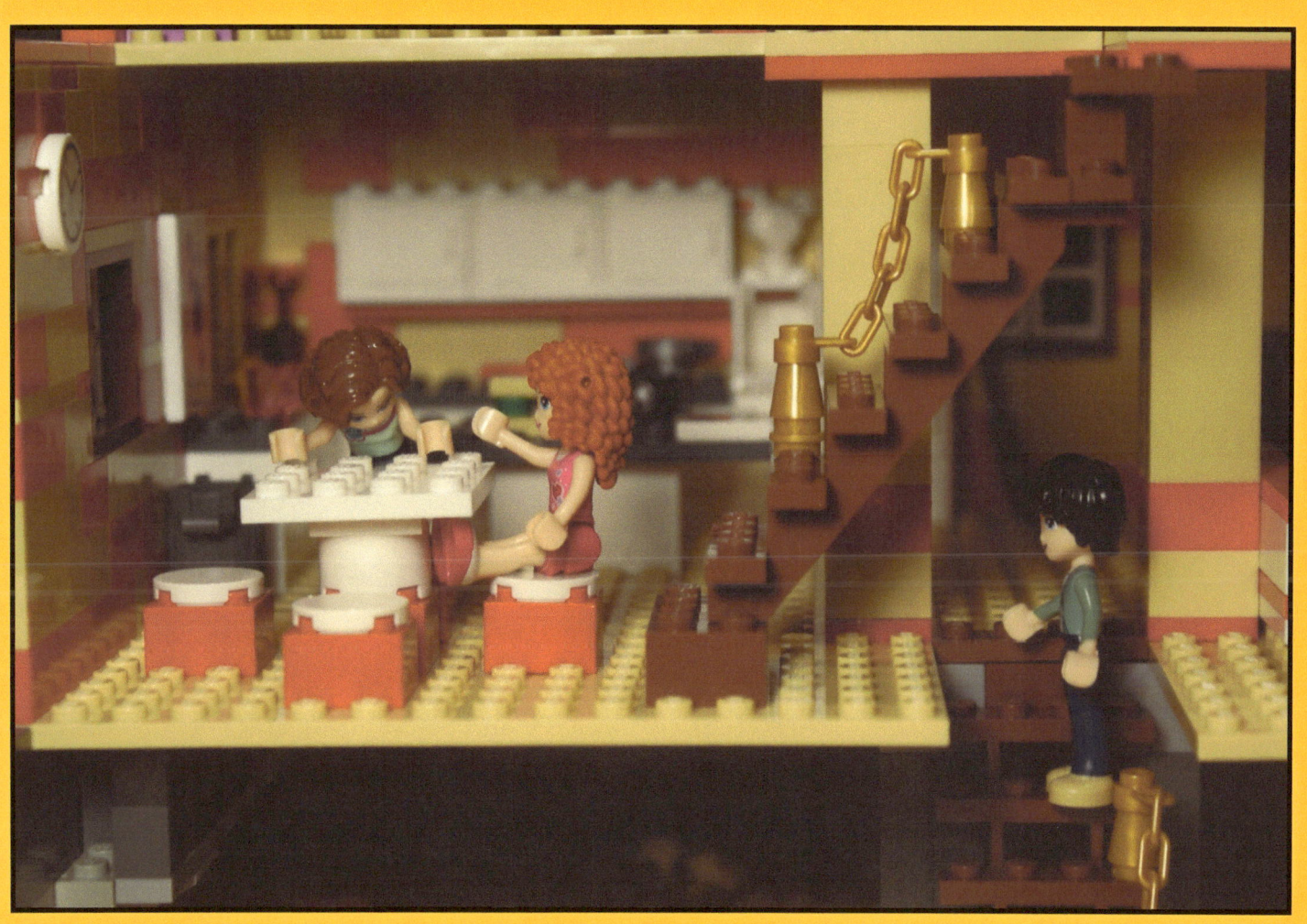

About the Author

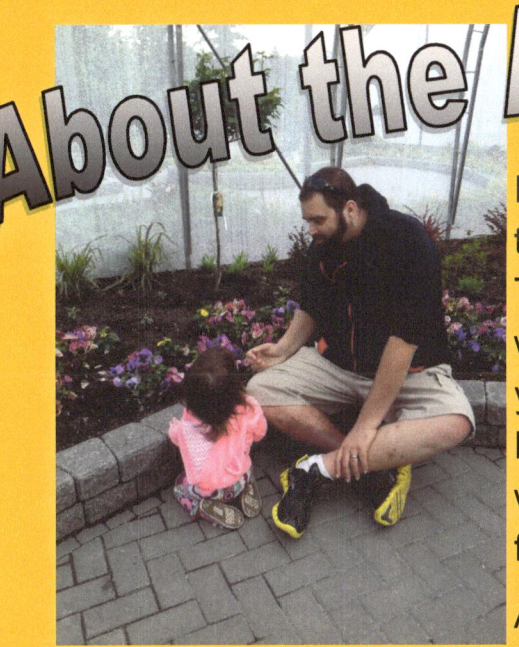

Amanda Stock is the author and photographer of Sometimes Mommy Falls and the upcoming books in the Talking to Kids about Narcolepsy series. These books were written to assist adults with explaining what Narcolepsy is to a young child or other people in their life. Having a young daughter, Amanda knew this would be an obstacle she would one day face and set out to find a solution.

Amanda is a wife and mother living with Narcolepsy. Like most Narcoleptics she began showing symptoms at age 15 but was not diagnosed unto age 26. Receiving that diagnosis was a huge relief. Understanding what the problem was and how to manage it has made a big difference in her life.

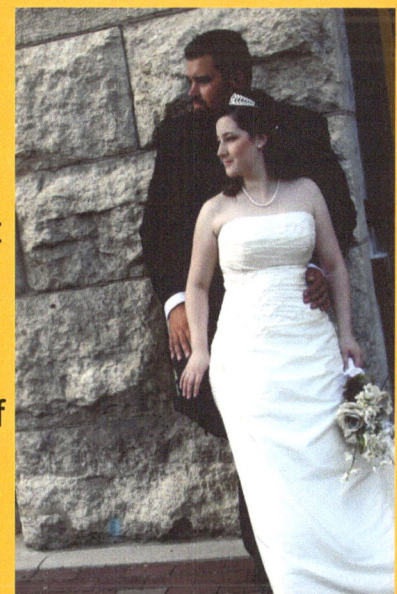

The Talking to Kids about Narcolepsy book series has been a three year project due to the author's incredible lack of drawing skills. This book series is in no way